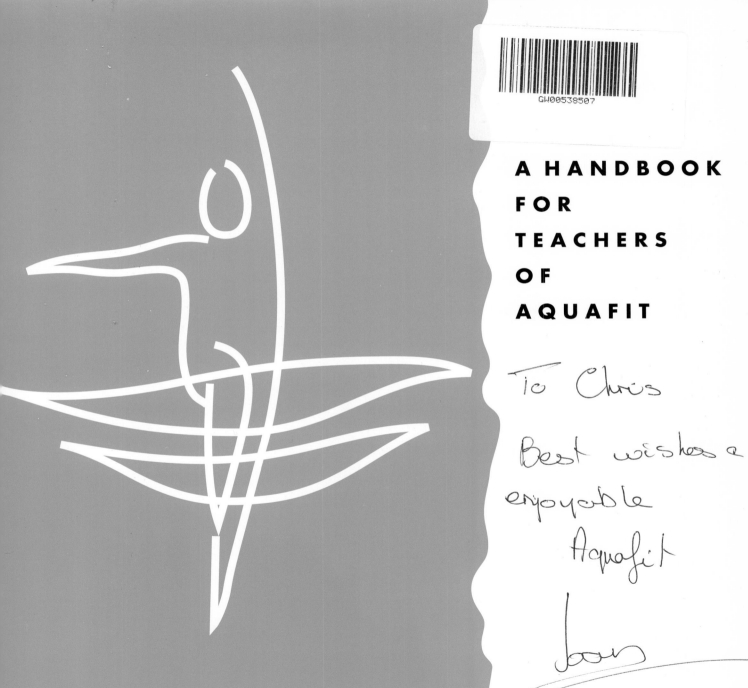

A HANDBOOK FOR TEACHERS OF AQUAFIT

To Chris

Best wishes a
enjoyable
Aquafit

Acknowledgements

To Peter and Anne for their help in the initial preparation of the handbook.
To the University Swim Centre and Marketing Services, Corporate Affairs
Department for the final preparation.

With the co-operation of the Amateur Swimming Association.

Copies of this book are available from The Swim Centre, University of Sunderland.
Tel 091 5152937.

First published 1991
Second (revised) edition 1993
© Copyright University of Sunderland
ISBN 1 873757 01 8 Teaching Aquafit: A Handbook for Teachers of Aquafit. (2r.e.)
Published by the University of Sunderland

This book was designed and produced by Marketing Services, Corporate Affairs
Department.

Contents

Introduction

This booklet is written to help all tutors, teachers and aspiring teachers of aquafit (exercise to music in water). Having taught aquafit over 10 years and run many teacher training courses I have collected information which I hope this booklet presents in a logical way. It may be used as a supporting text for those attending an aquafit teachers' course and as a subsequent source of reference.

This booklet does not set out exercises in detail but gives the knowledge which is required to plan exercise programmes. The aquafit courses for teachers give examples of exercises to use and all teachers will develop their own exercises through working in water themselves.

This book is a set of guidelines to assist in the planning and teaching of water exercise classes and to encourage high standards of safety and class care. Teachers of aquafit must be well informed to work responsibly and to set up safe and enjoyable classes. Participants should benefit from the classes and wish to continue.

Why Exercise in Water?

Why exercise?

Regular participation in water exercise is recommended to improve one's quality of life by improving health and fitness. The World Health Organisation defines good health as 'a complete feeling of mental and physical well being - not merely the absence of disease and infirmity, but the presence of vigour, vitality and social well being - a zest for living'.

Fitness is defined by the W.H.O. as the 'ability to carry out daily tasks with vigour and alertness without undue fatigue, with ample reserve energy to enjoy leisure pursuits and meet unforeseen circumstances'.

It is this fitness for life that aquafit is planned to promote. In common with other forms of exercise it aims to maintain or improve:

Suppleness Strength *and* Stamina
to reduce Stress
and to have Sociological *benefits*

These factors can be fulfilled through a well taught exercise session on land so - why in water?

Advantages and Effectiveness of Exercise in Water

Most problems with exercise programmes have arisen from strenuous routines with high impact work such as jogging and jumping. Good teachers of exercise are now very aware of potentially harmful situations arising and they teach with safety in mind. Exercising in water reduces the risks of injury providing the teacher plans a safe programme and is aware of individual needs.

It is the water which gives the safe medium for exercise and gives some unique benefits to this form of exercise session.

1. Water is friendly and offers an enjoyable medium in which to work.
2. Once the body is in the water it is virtually weightless. This makes movement easier for everybody, movements can be taken further. This fact is particularly important for people who are overweight or have a physical disability with limited mobility.
3. The buoyancy of the water helps suppleness and encourages relaxation.
4. Participants can work at the level which suits them. The water offers resistance which can be used

to make movements easier or harder.

5. Above all exercise in water is safe, there is little chance of straining muscles or damaging joints. Water cushions the body, so protecting the spine from damage.

6. The movement of the water around the body mass which is below the water surface gives a massaging effect. This helps to tone and shape the body.

7. It is possible to work hard without overheating the body, it is unusual to sweat whilst exercising in water.

8. When working in water participants have to think about breathing, the pressure of water around the thorax makes it harder to breathe.

9. Exercise in water is a very comfortable and enjoyable way of getting fit, it eases fatigue, helps relaxation and gives a good feeling when the session is finished.

This should be a form of exercise without pain or strain, it is a safe form of exercise. It is possible to plan and teach sessions to meet varied fitness levels. To make exercise in water effective it is necessary to understand the unique properties of water and apply them to the exercise programme.

Buoyancy

The buoyancy of water makes the submerged part of a person's body 90% lighter than on land. It is buoyancy which makes exercise in water safer.

1. It reduces compression stress on weightbearing joints, bones and muscles, so eliminating injury from impact as when running or jumping.

2. The cushioning effect protects the body from uncontrolled movements which may damage joints or strain muscles.

3. Buoyancy can make movements easier and increase the range of movement possible in a joint. Try standing on land, lift one leg as high as possible and hold it for a minute or longer. Then try the same in water, the water lifts your leg higher and makes it easier to hold the position. This enables people with painful joints to take a movement further without pain. Water buoyancy encourages a fuller range of movement in a joint, so improving suppleness.

4. The density of the human body varies according to the relative proportion of fat and muscle. This variation will be evident in any class. Teachers must adapt their teaching to accommodate this variation. It may be necessary to use different starting positions. Less buoyant people may need a float between their legs for some floating type exercises. Those with greater buoyancy may need to work

in shallower water for standing exercises in order to keep contact with the pool floor. They should find a floating position easy but one requiring the hips to be in towards the pool wall very difficult.

5. Water cushions the body in a supported position so protecting the spine.

6. The virtual weightlessness makes water a suitable and safe exercise medium for antenatal groups, the overweight and those with physical disabilities. It facilitates movement that these people may not normally be able to perform on land.

7. Teachers must always consider the depth of water being used for various exercises. When submerged only to the waist gravitational pull is only reduced to 50%. This additional weight out of the water may help for some exercises but can increase the strain on the body.

8. Buoyancy gives good body support but those participants not used to being in water do not automatically adjust to the water movement. Help must be given to aid this balance by:

a) teaching the correct starting position. When standing, bent knees help to lower the base and give a firmer position.

b) checking the depth of water for each individual.

c) teaching how to use the arms and hands to aid balance by a sculling type movement. This is particularly important for leg exercises and aerobic work.

Resistance

As the body or limbs move through water the resistance set up causes drag. Swimmers try to streamline the body to reduce resistance but then use the resistance to give propulsion. In aquafit the drag effect when exercising in water strengthens the muscles. The resistance is directly related to the speed and effort of the movement. Doubling the speed of a movement quadruples the resistance. The strengthening effect depends on the effort made, the speed of the movement and the surface area presented to the water.

When working in water every movement must be initiated by the muscles as gravity does not assist. The muscle action is concentric action as limbs are not held against gravity. There is little eccentric action. This factor eliminates most of the stiffness frequently experienced following a land based class. Teachers must understand how to use the resistance of the water and explain this to their class. Indicate where the most effort is to come in a movement according to the muscle groups to be worked. The body parts mainly being exercised should be submerged. This should be checked, particularly in arm work. The effort can be varied for each individual according to the speed of the movement and the sheer power exerted on the water. Resistance can be increased by the use of paddles. This increases the toning effect. Teachers must judge when paddles should be used and not necessarily by the whole class. Many benefits of exercise in water are lost if the teacher does not encourage effort in the movement and check that individuals understand how to use the water to maximum effect. Buoyancy and resistance together enable individuals to work within their own ability and at their own pace.

Water Temperature

 The temperature of the water and the air in the building is important, but there is probably little the teacher can do about it. An ideal temperature is about 86 degrees with the air temperature slightly higher. The teacher must try to keep the participants comfortably warm throughout the session. A water temperature of about 86 degrees allows a continuous period of hard strenuous exercise to be taken without any discomfort from overheating and little sweating. Initial immersion in water causes a drop in the body temperature. This makes the warm up important.

1. As soon as individuals enter the water encourage them to immerse their body and to move.
2. Keep up the pace of the lesson by using warming breaks between slower or static exercise routines.
3. Watch out for signs of cold, tenseness, shivering, poorly coordinated movements. Change the activity if necessary.
4. A shorter session with continuous activity is much better than a longer session with static breaks.
5. Elderly people may need only a 20 minute session if the water is cooler than 86 degrees. Similarly for antenatal groups or those with physical disability.
6. Exercise in water which is too warm means that the heat transfer from the body to the water cannot take place and this can lead to fatigue and heat exhaustion, just like exercising on a hot day. This can occur in a hydrotherapy pool, a facility which is not normally suitable for classes but which may be needed for those with physical disability.

Water Movement

 To be immersed in water can be a very pleasurable experience. It can encourage relaxation and reduce stress. The movement of the water creates a body massage. It is a discreet environment in which to exercise. Participants are hidden from public view and are less conscious of their bodies once they are immersed.

 Teachers should encourage floating, sculling and slower movement, particularly in the cool down component. Breathing out into the water can encourage rhythmical and deep breathing and relaxation. Water is a friendly medium, classes should be enjoyable, participants should laugh and let off steam although they are working. They should enjoy moving in water.

Cardio-Vascular Fitness, The Effects of Water

For any exercise programme to develop cardio-vascular (cardio-respiratory) fitness it must have aerobic activities. When working on land it is fairly easy to monitor the heart rate. Hard exercise results in rapid and deeper breathing, feeling hot and sweating, and causing a more rapid heart beat. These factors are not so evident when exercising in water.

1. In water the heat from the body is dissipated very effectively. This results in a lower heart rate for the same amount of exercise. This can be beneficial as it enables exercise to continue without discomfort.
2. The cooler the water the lower will be the heart rate.
3. The reduced effect of gravity on the body immersed in water is thought to facilitate the return of blood to the heart. This may also reduce the heart rate and stress on the heart.
4. These factors mean that to raise the heart rate when in water requires harder work. But is also means that for certain specialist groups: antenatal,elderly, physically disabled, post-operative the lower heart rate whilst exercising may be an advantage.

Teachers should understand the principle of heart rate monitoring which is detailed in many physiology and exercise books. By working in the water themselves and monitoring their heart rate, teachers can understand the amount of work required to raise the heart rate. They will also appreciate the importance of the warm up section and the necessity for warming up activities throughout the session to try to maintain a heart rate level.

Although it is difficult accurately to monitor the heart rate when in water it nevertheless can give a useful guide to the intensity of the work. The heart rate falls quite quickly even in water at a temperature of 86 degrees and the cooler the water the more rapidly it falls.

A very simple formula can be used.
1. Take the heart rate over 6 seconds, beginning with zero. Multiply the answer by 10.
2. A level 1 group - those first starting to exercise, older people, antenatal groups, those just returning to exercise - should work at 60% to 70% of the maximum heart rate - 200.
3. A level 2 group - those who have been progressively exercising and are ready for harder work - 70% to 75% of maximum heart rate - 220.

4. A level 3 group - those with a good level of fitness already and with no physical contra-indications - 75% to 85% of maximum heart rate - 220.

Examples of the Formula

Maximum Heart Rate (Max H.R.) = 200 minus age.

40 year old - level 1
Max HR = 200-40 = 160
160 @ 60% = 96
160 @ 70% = 112
The recommended work rate would then be between
96 and 112 according to the progression through
a series of exercise sessions.

Maximum Heart Rate (MaxH.R.) = 220 minus age

30 year old - level 3
Max HR = 220-30 = 190
190 @ 75% = 143
190 @ 85% = 162
The working band in this case would be between 143 and 162.

Intensity, Frequency

1. To have any beneficial cardio-vascular effect the teacher must gauge carefully the intensity of the programme, gradually increasing this to give progression. Be particularly aware that level 1 participants must not be subjected to a hard aerobic session but must still raise the heart rate to the recommended level.

2. Encourage participants to take regular exercise such as walking, cycling, swimming as well as aquafit so they exercise 3 to 5 times a week. This frequency is necessary for a positive improvement.

3. Monitor the length of a session. It should last for at least 20 minutes. A 30 minute session is a good average for continuous work. The level 3 group can take a longer session.

4. Keep a work rate throughout the session. There should be no sudden stopping of activity. If participants feel tired they may need to reduce the level of work or change their activity but they should continue to be active even if just continuing with light jogging on the spot or sculling.

Safety Factors

1. The normal safety procedures applicable in a pool i.e. life guarding, safety equipment, and rules for hygiene in the pool area should apply.

2. An aquafit teacher should be a qualified life saver and be fully conversant with the health and safety procedures in any pool in which he/she is teaching.

3. Participants should not wear jewellery. This includes ear-rings and watches as quite serious accidents can be caused by hitting someone or inadvertently latching on to someone.

4. Long hair can be dangerous. Teachers should encourage participants to wear swimming caps or to tie their hair back.

5. In any class, all participants must be able to be seen and helped individually by the teacher. The popularity of these classes sometimes results in excessively large numbers. This can be dangerous and there is little chance of individual teaching or free movement. A guide may be a maximum of 20 to 30 in a class depending on the space available.

6. The teacher must work from the pool side so the class can be constantly under observation and the participants can see clearly the demonstrations. The teacher should be able to move freely around the pool side to quietly give individual help.

7. The teacher should adapt his/her teaching to fit the pool environment. Consider carefully the depth of the pool and the gradient. Is it a gentle or steep incline? On travelling activities is it safer for participants to move across the pool or lengthways? How suitable is the pool side for supported positions?

8. Be aware of non-swimmers. By using arm bands they can be helped to participate freely and safely in all activities. Ensure they are always safe.

9. Before starting any movement check the class is well spaced out. There is a tendency sometimes to crowd together or to stand in lines. Encourage the use of free space where everyone has room to exercise without danger. Constantly check that free standing or floating exercises are performed a safe distance from the pool wall.

10. Check that the depth of water is suitable for the exercise and the height of the participant.

Level of Group. Planning for participants of a similar level to form a group gives a safer working situation and usually a more harmonious feeling. It is advisable to have separate antenatal and 50+ groups. A level 3 fit group gives the opportunity for a high intensity class.

Screening. It is advisable to have some screening before starting the class through a well constructed and discreet application form. A teacher needs to know: swimming ability, any sight or hearing problems, any hidden disabilities such as epilepsy, asthma, cardiac problems, arthritic conditions, replacement hips, back problems and any post-operative patients. Pregnant and elderly participants should seek medical approval before starting any exercise course.

Pool Side. The pool side can be a dangerous place for the teacher when demonstrating exercises. If the side is very slippery it may be necessary to use an area covered by a non-slip mat. Whilst jogging and jumping on the poolside the teacher may need to wear cushioning non slip footwear.

Tape Recorder. This must be plugged into a circuit breaker or as a safer option used with batteries. Avoid touching the machine with wet hands.

Exercise Safety. The correct planning and teaching of exercise is essential to avoid injury. This is covered in the section on planning sessions.

Facilities and Equipment

1. Pool. Ideally a pool with a largish area of shallow water - 1 to 1.5 metres in depth and with a deep water section. Learner pools or all over very shallow pools are not suitable.
Trough, rail or pool side suitable for support. A pool side on which the teacher can move around easily whilst keeping the class in view.
Temperature approximately 86 degrees or warmer.

2. Equipment. Hand paddles
Floats - 2 per participant
Balls - medium size
Long poles or hoops
Wrist/ankle weights for toning (level 3 groups)
Arm bands or other flotation aid

3. Tape Recorder. With good volume and a variety of taped music.

4. Dress. Participants need a well fitting swim suit/trunks. For women swim suits with a higher neck line give better support. A supportive bra or minimum bounce bra with a T-shirt may be preferred by some participants. The teacher should be neatly attired in a way that allows the participants to see all movements clearly. Shorts, tights with leotard or support top, swim suit and short sleeved top, some teachers may need a good bra support.

The Structure of an Aquafit Session

The design and structure of the programme reflects the aims of the work. Any session should give class members a good general workout aiming to improve stamina, strength and suppleness but also be concerned with emotional fitness. It should be enjoyable and there should be a good class atmosphere with a sense of belonging to a group. Encourage a happy feeling.

Every session should include the following components:
Warm Up
Muscular Strength and Endurance
Aerobic/Stamina
Cool Down

Normally I use this order in the planning as I find when working in water if aerobics follow warm up the second half of the session tends to become more static and does not build to a climax. The cooling effect of the water requires constant resort to warming activities. In the strength and endurance section it may be necessary to include linked warming breaks. However, the placing of the components within a session may vary, the structure and emphasis should reflect the fitness levels of the participants and the specific aim of a session.

Warm Up

This must start every session as it prepares the body for more demanding work. A warm up is necessary before any form of exercise to reduce the risk of injury.
A warm up should:
1. Increase the blood flow
2. Increase the body temperature
3. Increase the muscle elasticity
4. Decrease the muscle viscosity so increasing its mechanical efficiency
5. Increase the range of movement of the joints through an increase in the supply of synovial fluid to the joints and so reduce the wear and tear on joints
6. Gradually accelerate the cardio-vascular system
7. Contribute to better exercise performance in the subsequent aspects of the session as the body has already rehearsed exercise patterns

As the mind has been focussed on body exercise the participant is more ready to concentrate on the subsequent exercise programme.

To fulfil these aims a warm up should include the following:

1. Movements that are easy to follow so there is no delay in starting and no need to stop the flow of the sequence
2. Movements that will gradually raise the heart rate and the body temperature
3. Exercises that gently mobilise and loosen the whole body
4. Static stretching exercises
5. The warm up should be a continuous period of exercise lasting 5 - 8 minutes with a balance of rhythmic warming and mobilising exercises interspersed with static stretching exercises

Planning and Teaching the Warm Up

1. Start the participants as soon as they are in the water, be sure they are really 'wet' at least to above the shoulders or they will tend to work with tension in the upper body.
2. Plan warming exercises which are easy to follow. These exercises need to use large muscle groups and involve movement. Walking, running, jumping, swaying. A core of selected locomotor exercises can be repeated. The movements should not be too fast or intense. They need to be large movements moderately paced to gradually increase the heart rate. Nevertheless they should be sufficiently energetic to warm the body. Increase the intensity of work gradually through this section.
3. Mobility exercises should be interspersed between the warming movements. Concentrate on specific joints working in their full range of movement. The movements should be generally large, not too fast, at this stage concentrating on extent of movement in the joints rather than on powerful actions. Work through the body systematically.

Movements may include:

Ankle - ankle circling

Knees - standing knees bend and stretch. Lift one leg holding just above the knee bend and stretch the lower leg.

Hip - standing draw circle on pool floor, forward, side, back.

Lower Back - standing, knees slightly bent, pelvic circles.

Waist - standing, side bend, bend knee slightly into the bend.

　　　　- standing, arms held out in front, swaying movement to give side to side twist. Keep hips facing forward.

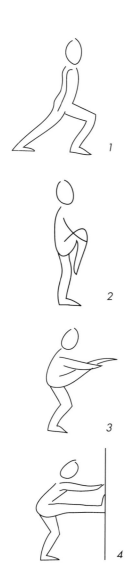

Basic Stretches

Shoulders and shoulder girdle - standing, shoulders under the water, shoulder rolls
- standing, bringing shoulders forwards and backwards, raising and lowering
- standing, hands to shoulders, circle elbows.
Elbows - standing - shoulders under the water, elbow bending and stretching.
Hands, Wrists - wrist circling
- finger bend, stretch and wriggle.
Develop your own repertoire of mobilising exercises which you can use.

Stretching Exercises

1. Stretching exercises should be taken after the muscles have been warmed, this places them normally in the second half of the warm up component.
2. Move into the stretch position slowly and hold the position for 5 - 10 seconds. There must be no forcing or bouncing.
3. Encourage easing a stretch out further after the initial stretch has been achieved.
4. The stretch should be felt in the belly of the muscle being stretched.
5. The buoyancy of the water makes it harder to feel a stretch than when performed on land.
6. Aim to stretch all the major muscles groups and to have a feel of stretch throughout the body. The stretch must be slow. If it is performed quickly or jerkily the stretch reflex muscle contraction will inhibit the movement. When a stretch is held the tension in the muscle relaxes and the stretch can be taken further.
7. Teach the stretches carefully and observe that the performance is correct - the extent of the stretch will vary according to the flexibility of each individual.

Basic Stretches

By trying movements yourself in water you will find other starting positions and stretches that can be used.

Calf stretch
In a forward lunge position with the toes of the back foot forward, press the heel down. (1)

Hamstring stretch
Standing, bring one knee up high to the chest and hold, use the arms to bring the knee high.(2)

Stand on one leg, bend the supporting leg, with the hands behind the thigh raise the other leg as high as possible (a more advanced stretch).(3)

Calf and Hamstring
At the wall, bend the supporting leg and take the other leg to a support on the wall, foot flat, lean forwards towards the leg, hands to the wall. (4)

Quadriceps
Stand, take one leg back to bring the heel to the seat, hold the foot. (5)

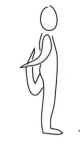

Groin
Stand - slide one leg out sideways, let the other knee bend. This can be taken on to a sideways leg lift, and a body dip sideways.(6)

Shoulder Stretch
Stand, reach up high with both arms, stomach pulled in. Take alternate arms into a slow high stretch. Feel the pull down the side of the body.

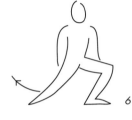

Spine
Sideways lunge position, stretch over to one side, keep facing front, lower hand on to knee. (7)
Stand feet astride, clasp both hands together in front on the water, slowly twist, let the knees give, hold the twist. (8)

In all stretches let the head follow the movement rather than taking any isolated cervical spine stretches.

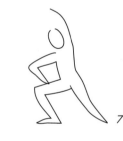

Muscular Strength and Endurance

In this part of the session isotonic exercise is used. This is dynamic moving exercise which develops strength throughout the body and through the full range of movement. When working in water concentric contraction of the muscle is used against the resistance of the water, this is a shortening of the muscle. When working on land the muscles are also used to control the body against gravity giving eccentric work, a lengthening of the muscle. It is the eccentric work which tends to give stiffness after a workout. Participants rarely suffer muscle soreness following an aquafit session, as there is virtually no eccentric muscle work.

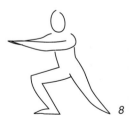

Basic Stretches

In the M.S.E. section you aim to:

1. Improve or maintain the strength of the muscles. This should improve muscle tone which should help in holding a good posture and in firming the body to give a good body shape.

2. Improve muscular endurance enabling the body to continue to work over a longer period of time without fatigue. To meet these aims movements should take place under the water.

Planning the M.S.E. Component

1. To improve muscle strength it is necessary to work hard against the resistance of the water. In each exercise plan when and how power is to be applied for the desired effect on the body.

2. Select a suitable starting position. In any lesson a variety of starting positions should be used. Check the teaching points you will use to achieve a correct position (refer to notes on posture/pelvic tilt).

3. Select and work yourself through 2 to 4 exercises for selected muscle groups or an area of the body. A routine for the legs/hips to strengthen mainly quadriceps, hamstrings, adductor and abductor muscles might be:

a) standing at the rail - leg swing forward and back

b) standing at the rail - leg stretch sideways and across to the wall

c) face the wall - legs astride, bounce up and down, heels down each time, good stretch on push up. Turn and repeat using the other leg.

Plan several repeats of each exercise and repetitions of the whole routine. The number of repetitions planned and the speed of the work will depend on the fitness of the group.

4. When planning a routine make it easy to change from one exercise to the next. If using apparatus, paddles or balls use them for the whole routine.

5. In each lesson try to plan a routine for each area of the body, and the muscle groups working the joints of that body area. Normally plan three M.S.E. routines:

a) for the upper body - arms and shoulder girdle

b) for the middle - spine, abdominal and back muscles

c) for the lower body - legs and pelvic area

6. Select appropriate music to accompany routines.

Teaching the M.S.E. Component

1. When introducing a new routine teach slowly and clearly and without music to ensure the aim of the exercises and the way to perform them are understood.

a) Ensure the starting position is correct and comfortable for all individuals. Check on good posture and on a suitable depth of water.

b) Teach through demonstration and give teaching points for the exercises of the routine. Put emphasis on how the power is to be used to utilise the water resistance.

c) Add the music, use cues and demonstration to lead the routine.

d) Give group and individual teaching points.

2. Observe the group to check on correct performance, and the maintenance of the starting position to give a firm base for the exercise. Check also that the speed and intensity of the work is suitable for the group.

3. If the water is cool or a routine has been rather static or slow follow with a more energetic break to keep up the heart rate and warm the body. The break should use the part of the body which has just been working - running or leg kicking on a float following leg exercises.

4. When you are demonstrating on the pool side be mobile, select a position where the group can see you clearly. This must be planned carefully when the participants are working at the rail, if they turn to face the opposite direction it will be necessary to change your teaching position. The class must be able to see you without twisting; this may disturb their starting position.

5. Over a series of lessons it is necessary to progress the work to overload the muscles and so improve strength. This may be done in the following ways:

a) Encourage harder work, more power as required by each exercise to work the selected muscles. Faster work.

b) Increase the resistance by using floats or hand paddles (level 2 or 3).

c) Add ankle or wrist weights (level 3).

6. To progress the endurance aspect increase the number of repetitions of each exercise and the repetitions of a routine.

7. The decision to progress work must reflect the ability and fitness level of the group and of individuals.

8. Progression in power, rate or repetitions may not be appropriate for some level 1 groups. For them the mobility of the body may be more important, requiring slower full range movements with power applied only as suitable to individuals.

For the M.S.E. component good posture and starting positions are essential for effective exercise.

Posture - Pelvic Tilt

In every starting position remind participants to assume a good posture. A feeling of flattening the back (lumber spine) and lengthening the body so extending the spine. Help to gain the correct pelvic tilt by teaching it when standing:

   Stand with feet slightly apart, knees slightly bent, toes facing forward.

Tighten abdominal muscles and muscles of the buttocks. Tuck the pelvis under (like tipping a basin). This should flatten the lumbar spine. This practice can be taken with the back to the pool wall to feel the position, press the lumbar spine to the wall.

   The teacher should constantly give reminders of correct posture. This applies to lying as well as to standing positions.

Starting Positions

1. Standing in a free space
a) Standing feet astride
b) Standing one foot in front of the other
Used for lower limb and arm exercises. When working arms a more stable base is achieved by standing in waist deep water and bending the knees to lower the centre of gravity. The abdominal muscles must be used strongly to stabilise the position and flatten the back and give a firm position for exercise.

The feet must grip the pool floor and constantly adjust to give good balance to the body. When standing and performing leg exercises the arms should be in the water using a sculling type movement to retain body balance. For participants unused to balancing in water guidance in retaining a stable position will be necessary.

2. Standing at the pool side
a) Side to wall
b) Face to wall
c) Back to wall
The wall assists balance and gives a stable position for strong leg work. The body should show good posture and remain stable so the main movement is restricted to the legs. Participants may find one hold easier than another, so encourage them to experiment and select a hold which helps them to carry out the exercise successfully.

3. Supported at the pool side
a) Front lying - hold one hand above the other or hands level.

b) Back lying or back sitting - hold with the arms extended sideways along the trough or pool wall, or with the elbows bent with a grip on the wall/trough close to the ears. The head may be lifted or lie back on the water. Decide whether the exercise is best performed in the lying or sitting (back against the wall) position.

c) Side lying - one hand grips the trough or wall, one hand pushes against the wall.

d) Suspended vertically - this can be taken facing or with the back to the wall, in deep water so the legs are free to move.

e) Foot support - feet are hooked under a rail or round the smooth side-supports of the steps.

All these support positions are useful for working the leg muscles and abdominals. 3 a) and b) are easier than the other positions but participants need to find a suitable hold to suit their buoyancy and shoulder flexibility.

4. Floating with floatation aids

Horizontal front, back, side and vertical floating and gliding positions with a float under each hand, or a ball or float held close to the body or stretched above the head. These give comfortable lying positions for most people and changing from one float or glide position to another is an exercise in itself. Leg, abdominal and arm exercises can be taken from these floating positions. The vertical float can give a base for strong leg work and abdominal work. Non-swimmers may wear arm bands to help the maintenance of a floating position.

5. Sculling

Swimmers who are competent at sculling can hold the previous floating positions using sculling. This gives strong arm work as well as the designated leg or abdominal work but be sure the effort is put into the exercise to effect the selected muscles and not mainly into the sculling.

6. Partner support

Partner supports may be used for floating positions taking the support under the shoulder blades when lying on the back and as an elbow or shoulder support on the front. Suggest experimenting to achieve a comfortable position. This support is useful for less confident participants and is often a comfortable position for pregnant ladies.

7. By changing a starting position an exercise can be made easier or harder whilst using the same muscle groups.

Aerobic Component

Aims of this component

1. To provide a cardio-respiratory training effect by giving a period of exercise of the right intensity and duration for individuals and groups.
2. To improve the aerobic capacity, that is the ability to take up large amounts of oxygen, transport it efficiently through the blood stream and produce energy for work in the muscles.
3. To further warm up the body
4. To give an enjoyable and lively sequence of movements to music.

Effects of water

In order to achieve the appropriate training effect it is necessary to work really hard in water. This is necessary because of the cooling effect of water and the lack of gravitational pull on the body. To counteract this to some extent and to work safely when running and jumping the aerobic component is normally taken in waist deep water. Working in deep water (chest deep) can increase the effect for some travelling activities such as running. The wall of water in front of the body makes for harder work.

Swimming activities can be a valuable part of an aerobic section if the participants are sufficiently confident and skilful to maintain a level of performance.

Jumping type activities which for many people would not be safe on land can be used in water as there is no hard impact with the floor of the pool, buoyancy counteracts the landing force, the knees should give on landing.

It takes three times as much energy to walk in water as to walk on land making fast paced locomotion or other movements more fatiguing than on land.

Planning and Teaching the Aerobic Component

1. Consider the ability, age and fitness level of your group. This will effect the intensity and duration of your work.
2. Be aware of the water/air temperature.
3. Include movements using large muscle groups. Involve travelling, large jumping, running, hopping and stepping type movements.
Use large continuous body movements on the spot or travelling.
4. Do not make the routine too difficult to follow. Using a core of movement which is repeated as a

'chorus' gives known repetition before introducing a new movement and makes a sequence easier to follow.

5. When planning the routine remember movement in water is slower than on land unless the movements are very small.

6. If including change of direction or circling give time as these are harder to perform in water.

7. Take any movement long enough for it to be established before changing the movement.

8. Work out the aerobic routine yourself to the music preferably practising it on land then in the water to check that the speed of music is suitable and the movement changes are possible.

9. Start this component straight away to the music with your pool side demonstration and voice leading the routine. It is hard for a teacher working on the pool side so once a movement has been learnt the voice or an arm demonstration can be used to remind the participants of the action.

10. Partner work, group work, country dance style routines, ball work and swimming can all be used in aerobic routines.

11. Use the pool area freely. Encourage the use of the arms to help running and jumping. Participants may need guidance as to how to use their arms and hands to help balance and propulsion.

12. Although this component should involve hard work it should also be enjoyable. It is up to the teacher to set the right atmosphere through the music, the choice of routine and the lively presentation.

13. The aerobic component can last from 5 to 15 minutes depending upon the fitness level and ability of the group.

14. Checking the heart rate immediately after the aerobic component can give the teacher and the participant a guide to the level of work and the suitability of the intensity and duration.

Cool Down, Relaxation Component

Aims of this component:

1. To gradually return the body to the pre-exercise state.
2. To relax and reduce tension.
3. To stretch muscles at the end of the work out.
4. To calm the class down for the end of the session.

Planning and Teaching the Cool Down

1. Plan movements and exercises which gradually reduce the heart rate from the end of the aerobic component. Move more slowly, walk, scull and reduce the intensity of the work.

2. Take movements which are not working hard against the resistance of the water e.g.

a) Breathing, blowing bubbles

b) Bobbing movements

c) Free slow work with balls or hoops

d) Return to slow stretches as explained for the warm up. Move gently in and out of the stretches and hold 10 to 15 seconds.

e) Floating, changing shape and holding positions

f) Mobility work, take large slow mobility exercises

3. The body cools down quickly in water, beware of the participants becoming too cold.

4. This is a fairly short component, just long enough to achieve the aims.

5. Select music which is slow, easy to listen to and which encourages a flowing routine of movement.

6. Participants often enjoy the opportunity to work freely on a theme in this section e.g. circular movements, travelling, 'changing shape' composing a ball or hoop sequence.

General Teaching Method for an Aquafit Session

1. Prepare your programme content well, see there is variety in content, speed and the use of different starting positions. Include movement on the spot and travelling. Use pool equipment when applicable to add interest. Include partner and group work.

2. Prepare your music, use a variety of music to please all participants and to suit your routines.

3. Plan how you intend to introduce each component of a session, particularly when teaching new work.

4. Do teach, do not expect participants to observe and follow you accurately, verbal guidance will also be required.

5. Practise your demonstrations so you can perform them easily and accurately.

6. Adapt your work as you go through a session if the planned material seems too easy, too difficult or the water temperature is particularly cold or hot.

7. Encourage hard work, it is very easy to do the minimum when in water. The level of work you demand must suit the individuals.

8. Do remind participants to breathe as they work. Emphasise breathing out.

9. Progress and vary the content of a class to avoid the participants losing interest and not benefiting from the session.

10. Always work for good quality performance, do not just rush through a session. Explain how effort

is to be applied. Participants should, through repetition, improve the quality of their performance. They will then be ready to increase the intensity of the work.

11. Change the speed of a movement. An exercise may be taught and performed quite slowly in full range then by increasing the speed the intensity will be dramatically increased. Be sure this does not lead to 'cheating', reducing effort or range of movement. Change of speed in a routine also adds interest.

12. As progress is made the M.S.E. and aerobic components can be extended in time to increase the aerobic and endurance effects.

13. For adults to adhere to an exercise programme they must feel it is doing them good and they should enjoy participating and the atmosphere of the session. This is entirely up to the teacher. Variety, fun, good presentation and an effective exercise programme should encourage continued participation. If a teacher enjoys teaching aquafit, the class are likely to enjoy the sessions.

Chapter IV

The Aquafit
Session-Groupings

Aquafit Session Groupings

Level 1 - Beginner Group

Within this group may be anyone returning to exercise after several years, post-operative, post-natal and possibly a high percentage of non-swimmers. It should begin as a fairly gentle class with emphasis on suppleness, taking joints through the full range of movement. Exercises tend to be slower with a gradual increase in pressure against the water. Through a course of lessons there is an increase in the repetitions of M.S.E. exercises. The aerobic section is short, 3 to 5 minutes, gradually increase this as the group progresses. As this group may include a wide range of ages and abilities individuals must be encouraged to work with more or less vigour as appropriate to their level of fitness.

Level 2 - Intermediate Group

This should be offered as a progression on level 1, the rate of progress to this group will vary with individuals, some may never aspire to this level. Every component of the lesson tends to be longer. Greater emphasis is placed on varying the speed of exercises and on the power in each movement. The aerobic section is longer and may, if appropriate, include swimming and the use of part and whole stroke practices. Introduce equipment to increase resistance such as paddles and floats.

Level 3 - Advanced Level

The work should be continuous for the 30 to 45 minute session. Resistance is maximised and the teacher encourages maximum effort on all underwater movements. The aerobic component lasts 10 to 15 minutes. At this level circuits are a useful form of work as they offer self challenge. Games and hard swimming may be included. There is an increase in repetitions of sets of exercises and routines. There is an emphasis on body toning and on raising the heart rate to the training level and keeping it there for at least 20 minutes. Whilst a faster pace may be set for exercises and movements the pace should be varied. It is still necessary to take large strong movements as well as smaller vigorous movements.

Elderly Group

There is a great range of fitness in the elderly age range and individuals may join level 1, 2 or 3 classes. But offering classes for post-retirement, fifty plus or third age, whatever they may be called, gives a cohesive group which can be offered in the day time. The social aspect of such a group is important.

1. The teacher needs to be aware of individual medical conditions (see safety chapter) and make the appropriate exercise adjustments.

2. Movement in the water is generally slower, particularly in changing direction as some of the elderly may find balance difficult consequently they do not react quickly to change.

3. More work may be taken with rail support to aid balance particularly lower limb stretches and exercises.

4. Level 1 work is usually an appropriate level, the aerobic section should begin easily without too much strain on the body but with progression in content and length over a series of lessons.

5. Exercises for feet and hands should be included as this group may suffer from stiffness which can be helped by movement in water.

6. Posture is important, a good standing position helps to tone sagging muscles and promote general health.

7. Individually comfortable starting positions are used. Floating supported by floats may be more comfortable than using a support at the wall.

8. Whilst muscle strengthening is important the number of repetitions should only be gradually increased.

9. The exercises and the movements are usually taken at a slower pace with encouragement to take large movements. Progress can be made but it is slow and cautious. There should always be encouragement to develop power in pushing against the water.

10. Courses of lessons should start gently and gradually build to more strenuous and continuous activities.

11. It is important to include movements which make participants puff a little and raise the heart rate. Start with a very short and not too vigorous aerobic component and gradually progress.

12. Hip arthroplasty (replacement). Participants who have undergone this operation will have been advised which movements to avoid when exercising. The teacher should avoid movements which bring the leg across the body (adduction) or wide to the side (abduction), hip pivoting exercises, breaststroke type action, jumping with knees out or with twisting actions.

13. Avoid strain on the lumber spine, take care with any exercise causing the back to hollow. Work to flatten the lumbar spine, check on good posture in all starting positions.

14. Group and partner activities are often enjoyed.

15. Music should be selected to suit the age range.

16. The water temperature should ideally be 86 degrees. In colder water it may be necessary to shorten the session.

17. Encourage breathing and relaxation, particularly in the cool down.

Antenatal Group

Water offers an ideal medium for exercises for pregnant women. It helps relaxation and relieves aches and pains often associated with pregnancy. It is a discreet form of exercise. The exercise programme can aid concentration on the body's movements and on breathing whilst also improving strength and general fitness.

1. A midwife should be present at each session.
2. Participants exercise only as much as is comfortable, avoiding any strain. Teachers must be aware of the variance in capacity for work and the difference in problems at all stages of pregnancy.
3. Exercise is slow and steady without fast and jerky movements.
4. Participants should be aware of how the body carries out each exercise and breathing should fit into the movements. Concentrate on exhalation.
5. Stretches should only be taken as far as is comfortable.
6. Walking and running steps may be taken but energetic jumping and bouncing type movements should be avoided.
7. Upper body exercises to tone and strengthen upper body muscles should be included. Balls and hand paddles can be used as long as no strain is felt.
8. Include lower body exercises to strengthen the muscles of the thigh and groin and to increase suppleness in the hip joints. Foot mobilising work and lower leg strengthening. This section will include exercises at the rail, travelling leg kicks on floats, leg exercises suspended or floating.
9. In every session there should be pelvic floor contractions. These should be taken in the warm up and again in the cool down.
10. Abdominal work should include gentle abdominal toning but without twisting or side bends and no excessively strong work.
11. Concentrate on good posture particularly good abdominal tone and tipping the pelvis to flatten the lumbar spine.
12. Avoid any exercise which will place strain on the lower back.
13. Floating, sculling and swimming should be included. Individuals will choose to swim on their front, back or side according to which they feel is the most comfortable.
14. Breath holding and swimming under water should be avoided.
15. Individuals must work at their own level throughout and get out of the water or rest if they feel any strain or tiredness.
16. The gentle work of the cool down session can be extended to encourage breathing and relaxation.

17. The recti abdominis muscles which are normally joined down the centre of the abdomen may part in the latter half of the pregnancy. It is at this time that only gentler abdominal exercises should be performed. Until these muscles are rejoined after pregnancy there should be no heavy abdominal work. The time taken for the muscles to join varies with individuals.

18. The water temperature should be 86 degrees for antenatal classes.

Post-natal Group

1. Aquafit for post-natal begins at level 1. It should include initially only gentle abdominal work but still include posture exercises and pelvic floor contractions.

2. Gradually the emphasis will be on the regaining of muscle tone and progress will be quite rapid to a normal toning and stamina session at level 2 and then level 3.

Conclusion

Advertising aquafit classes for special groups gives the teacher the opportunity to teach a session at the appropriate level. The participants have a suitable work out and usually enjoy working with those of similar age and/or ability. Participants should be expected to enrol for a course of lessons. It is difficult for a teacher and for members of the class if there is a constant change of individuals. Joining a class part way through a course can be dangerous as progression will have been made. Obviously a more flexible approach is necessary for an antenatal group.

Chapter V
The Use of Music

Use of Music

Music should be an aid to exercise, aquafit is essentially a water exercise programme using music. The musical component can have a powerful influence for the participants. It can be motivating, enjoyable, make them want to exercise and make them feel good. Music can set the pace, rhythm and mood of a routine. Music can set a happy atmosphere and can integrate the class and teacher. Whilst music can contribute in many ways to the class it should never be a distraction or only a background. It should enhance performance. Care must be taken that the quality of movement does not suffer in the effort to fit the music or because the teacher or class become so engrossed in the music that they forget the movement quality.

Selection of Music

This is a difficult and lengthy task. It involves listening to all forms of music and assessing the suitability for exercise. The following points may help you:

1. Build up a catalogue of suitable music, listing the source, type of music, beat, speed, aspect of a session for which it may be applicable.
2. Movements in water are slower than on land. It may be necessary to use double the number of beats for an exercise. Remember this when planning a routine on land. If music is used with a fast beat it will demand 4 times the effort in water and the movement cannot then be maintained for long.
3. Select music appropriate to the age, ability and fitness of the class.
4. Have a variety of tempo and style of music in any one session.
5. There is a great variety of music available, current popular, country and western, theme music, big band, classical, jazz. Whatever is selected should have a constant beat through the piece or be in clear phrases. Vocals should not impinge upon the voice of the teacher.
6. The teacher should enjoy working to the music.
7. There should be a regular change of music through a course of lessons.
8. 2/4 and 4/4 rhythms are easy to use, they give 8 or 16 beat phrases which are suitable lengths for the repetition of an exercise.
9. Waltz or 3/4 may be used for general movement, arm exercises or cool down.

Preparing Music

1. Plan your movement or exercise sequence in relation to the ability of the class then select the music.
2. Listen to the music several times, establish the beat, count it or clap it. This establishes the regular beat: 1234/1234; 123/123; 12/12.
3. Count the music into regular 8 counts and record on paper the breakdown e.g. 32 sets of 8.
4. Listen again to group together the phrases of 8. Are there phrases which sound the same and are repeated e.g. AABCAABCAADE
ABCDE represent different phrases of the music. A is repeated regularly. A teacher may think of this giving a repetition in the movement.
5. Having analysed the music work the selected exercise routine to it.
6. Talk through the music as you move to bring out cue words which you will use when teaching. Examples of cue words: and forward; and legs apart; and alternate arms-----. This practice will help you to remember the sequence of work and phrasing of the music.
7. A piece of music with a steady rhythmic beat and melody throughout is easy to use. The teacher can change from one exercise to another in a routine at the end of any phrase in the music.

Music for Session Components

Warm Up. This music tends to set the tone for the lesson, and it should motivate the class to join in. Music should be easy to follow. If choreographing a warm up sequence, music that has clear phrasing with a 'chorus' can be used. Linking two bands of music to fit the length of a warm up can commence with music suitable for warming and mobilising and then change to give slower music for stretching, finishing with further warming phrases.

Muscular Strength and Endurance. The music used for the exercise sequences should have a steady beat to give a continuous rhythmic and melodic accompaniment. The tempo will relate to the fitness of the group. The speed of the music must fit the exercises.

Aerobic Component. The music for this section should be lively with a clear beat to encourage vigorous work. The music needs to keep the class going. It should be enjoyable. The speed and vigour must relate to the group. A level 1 group will work more slowly than a level 3. When planning an aerobic sequence do relate to the slower movements in water, particularly when encouraging big jumps or runs.

Cool Down. Slower music to accompany slow stretches, breathing, easy controlled movements and relaxation.

Teaching to Music

1. The warm up and the aerobic section are normally started straight away to the music, the class following the teacher's demonstration and voice cues.
2. The exercises which require clear teaching to ensure a correct and safe performance are usually introduced initially without music. Once the class knows the exercise routine the music is brought in and the teacher cues the changes and also gives teaching points.
3. At times a group of exercises may be taken without music, the teacher then sets the rhythm and keeps the class going by the use of the voice.
4. All the tracks to be used in one session may be recorded on to one tape, but this will need to be changed regularly. Alternatively single tapes may be used for different sections of the lesson. This allows the teacher to be more flexible in the use of tracks according to the needs of the class. The class must be given some active movement whilst the tape is being changed.

Conclusion

Whenever possible work in water yourself as you plan the routine to music or work in the pool with a willing colleague. Adapting to the slower speed of water exercise becomes easier with experience. Always observe your class to check if the rhythm you are setting is suitable for the majority of the group.

Movements in the Main Joints

This handbook does not attempt to detail the anatomy and physiology background theory with which every teacher of Aquafit should be conversant. There are many books which set out quite clearly the necessary information on anatomy and physiology.

Teachers should have a knowledge of:-

1. The circulatory and respiratory systems.
2. The skeleton, its make up and functions.
3. The classification and structure of the joints.
4. The movements possible in the joints.
5. The main muscles. The position of the muscles in the body and the action of the main muscle groups.

The following is a guide to the movements referred to in this book:

Flexion - bending or decreasing the angle between two bones (closing a joint).

Extension - stretching, increasing the angle between two bones (opening a joint).

Abduction - moving away from the centre line of the body.

Adduction - bringing towards the centre line of the body.

Elevation - raising, as in lifting the shoulders.

Depression - pulling down, as in pulling down the shoulders.

Lateral flexion - bending sideways in the spine, trunk or neck.

Rotation - pivoting the body part inwards or outwards around the long axis of the bone (rotating the arm).

Circumduction - a circular action, a combination of the movements possible in the joint (circling the arm).

In order to plan a session, particularly the Muscular Strength and Endurance component, a teacher should be conversant with how the muscles work to give movement in the joints.

1. A muscle passes over the joint on which it works.
2. To give movement it shortens (contracts).
3. Muscle groups work in opposite pairs e.g.

flexors - extensors of the hip; abductors - adductors of the hip

To understand how muscles work place a handkerchief or tape following the line of a muscle across

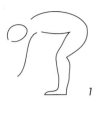

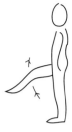

a joint, the tape will become slack (contract) as you perform the movement. The following table should help you to understand which muscles work to give the movements possible in the joints. As you follow the text try the movements on your own body.

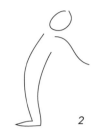

Movements in the Spine

Joints - between the vertebral bodies
1. Flexion - forward movement.
Abdominal muscles (rectus abdominis, internal and external obliques).
2. Extension - backward movement.
Long muscles of the back.
3. Lateral Flexion - side bending.
Abdominals (rectus abdominis) and back muscles of one side only.
4. Rotation twisting.
Abdominals (oblique muscles) back muscles.

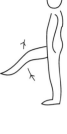

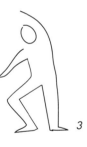

Movements in the Hip Joint

Hip joint, a ball and socket freely movable joint.
1. Flexion - leg moving forward towards body centre.
Hip flexors, iliopsoas, quadriceps, muscles at the front of the thigh and pelvis.
2. Extension - leg moves backwards.
Hip extension - gluteus maximus, hamstrings, muscles at the back of the thigh and buttocks.
3. Abduction - leg moves out sideways.
Abductors - muscles on the outside of the thigh.
4. Adduction - leg moves to centre and across the body.
Adductor muscles on the inside of the thigh.
5. Rotation - turning the leg inwards and outwards.
Combination of muscles acting on the hip joint.
6. Circumduction - circling the leg, a combination of all the above movements.

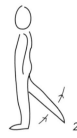

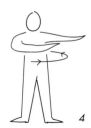

Movements in the Spine

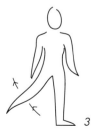

Movements in the Hip Joint

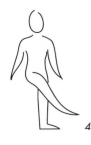

Knee joint

A hinge joint
1. Flexion - bend the knee, heel towards back of thigh. Hamstrings - muscles at the back of the thigh.
2. Extension - stretch the knee
Quadriceps - muscles at the front of the thigh.

Ankle Joint

A hinge joint
1. Dorsiflexion - bending the foot up towards the shin.
Tibialis Anterior - muscle at the front of the lower leg.
2. Plantor Flexion - extending the foot, pointing the foot.
Gastronemius - muscles at the back of the lower leg, the calf muscles.

The Shoulder Joint

A ball and socket freely movable joint.
1. Flexion - arm moves upwards in front of the body.
Muscles at the front of the shoulder joint and chest - deltoid and pectoral muscles.
2. Extension - arms moves backwards and upwards.
Muscles at the back of the shoulder joint and upper back - deltoid and latissimus dorsi.
3. Abduction - arm moves out sideways and upwards.
Muscles at the top of the shoulder joint - deltoid, supraspinatus.
4. Adduction - arm moves inward across the body.
Combination of muscles in front and behind the joint - pectorals and latissimus dorsi.
5. Rotation - turning the arm inwards and outwards.
Combination of muscles around the joint.
6. Circumduction - circling the arm, a combination of all the above movements and with all muscles around the joint involved.

Elbow Joint

Hinge joint.
1. Flexion - bending the lower arm, hand to shoulder.
Muscles at the front of the upper arm - biceps, brachialis.
2. Extension - stretching lower arm.
Muscles at the back of the upper arm - triceps.

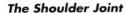

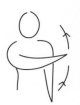

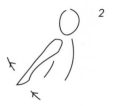

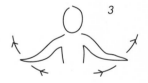

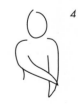

The Shoulder Joint

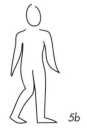

Further Reading

Aquafit - Shape Up the Safe & Effective Way
Harrison J. University of Sunderland Swim Centre 1993.

50+ a Safe Approach.
Fenham & Bassey. Sports Council Publication.

The English Y.M.C.A. Guide to Exercise to Music.
Callum R. & Mowbray L. Pelham Books 1988.

A Reference Manual for Teachers of Dance Exercise.
May J. Foulsham 1988.

Fitness for Life.
Corbin C.B. & Lindsey R. Scott, Foreman & Co. 1983.

Body in Action.
An introductory study pack.
Physiology and Performance.
Coaching handbook.
National Coaching Foundation.

Exercise Stop Danger.
British Australian Fitness Leader Network Publication.

Living Anatomy.
Connelly J. Human Kinetics.

Fitness For Sport.
Hazeldine R. Human Kinetics.

The Teaching of Swimming.
Amateur Swimming Association.

Synchronised Swimming.
Elkington H. & Chamberlin J. David & Charles.

Swimming Games and Activities.
Cregeen A. & Noble J. A& C Black. 1988.

Useful Addresses

For information on courses for teachers of exercise to music in water

1. The Amateur Swimming Association, Harold Fern House, Derby Square, Loughborough LE11 0AL.
2. The London Central Y.M.C.A. Training and Development Dept. 112, Great Russell Street, London, WC1B 3NQ.

Equipment for Aquafit
The Swim Shop, 52/58 Albert Road, Luton, Beds. LU1 3PR.

Books, Study Packs
1. The National Coaching Foundation, 4 College Close, Beckett Park, Leeds, LS6 3QH.
2. The Sports Council, 16 Upper Woburn Place, London, WC1H 0QP.
3. The Physical Education Association of Great Britain and Northern Ireland, 162 Kings Cross Road, London.

Video
An A.S.A. video is being prepared on the Teaching of Aquafit which will supplement this handbook.
For further information write to the A.S.A. Swimming Enterprises.

Music
Aquafit cassette, consisting of two sessions of music for exercise in water to accompany Joan Harrison's "Aquafit" book.
Available from University of Sunderland Swim Centre, Chester Road, Sunderland.